Forward

Many people suffer with unseen illnesses and debilitating diseases that cause them to withdraw from humanity itself. No healthy person genuinely expects their health will be taken away from them. For those that do not wish to withdraw from life and improve their physical condition, this book is dedicated to you.

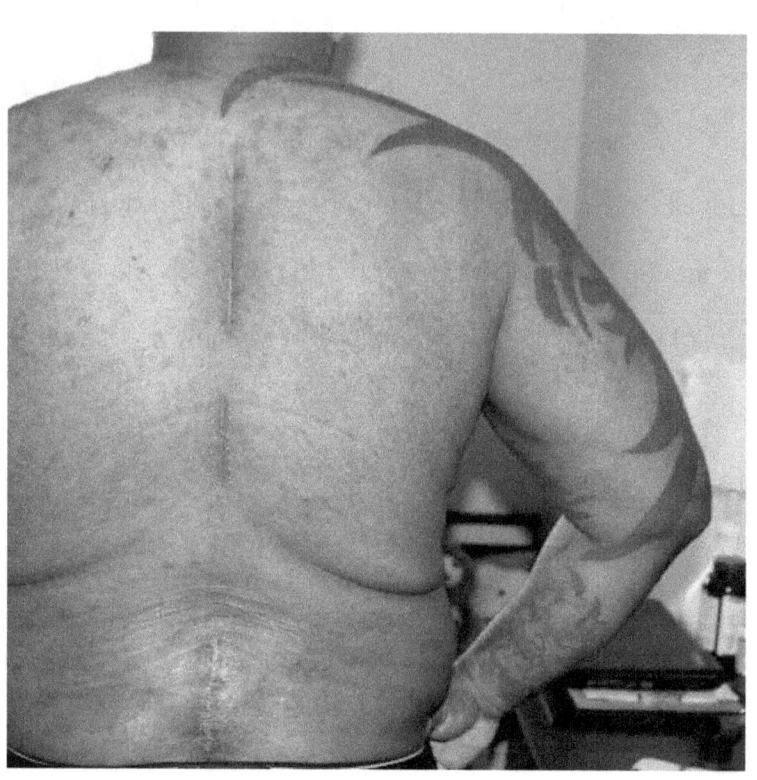

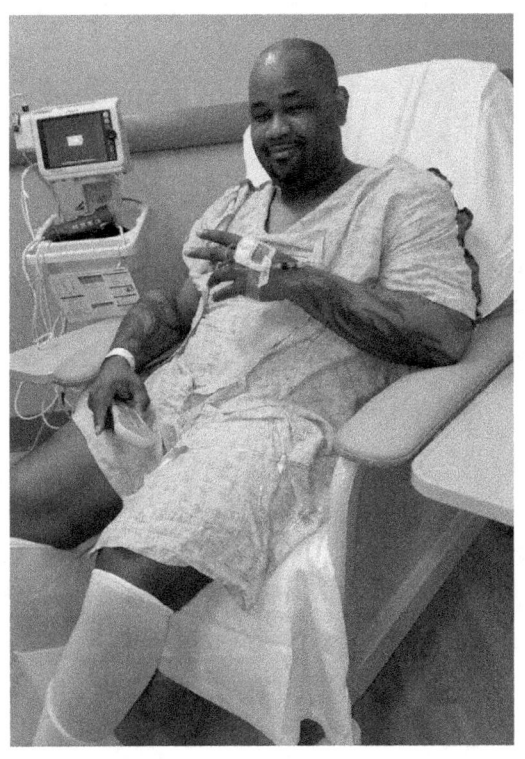

Author Dunneille Anderson (photo taken May 17, 2017 before a second back surgery)

THE SPINE FIX

BY DUNNEILLE ANDERSON

Introduction

If you are reading this you are probably a person that is very similar to myself, maybe you were a athlete that has sustained some type of back injury that has limited your life and you want to regain your life back. Maybe you are a person that wasn't an athlete but have a family to take care of and have sustained a debilitating back injury that has reduced your quality of life. Whomever you may be this book is for you, I wrote this book because I want people to know the truth about back surgery, recovery and the many pitfalls I faced while undergoing three severe back surgeries. I will detail in this book my experience, the lessons I have learned while rehabbing myself as well as what I have learned to change not only my physique but my general health as well. This book is designed to:

- Help you understand how to deal with your back injury/surgery mentally and physically
- Alleviate some of the fears of back surgery
- Help you to better understand how lifestyle effects your back
- Allow you to be a better version of what you were before
- Remove some of the frustrations of your injury and it's effect on your lifestyle by sharing my experience

Sports and Pain are Synonymous

Here is a little background regarding my back issues and diagnosis. I was a former athlete, I played football from junior high school thru college with a short stent as an arena football player. I also have a background in USA Boxing, Power Lifting, Muay Thai and MMA. As a youth playing sports I didn't experience too many injuries, the most severe injuries I had were a couple of ankle sprains and the typical football player shoulder strains. Well I should honestly say the only injuries that kept me off the field was those listed in the last sentence, but I had experienced pain in my mid-back beginning my junior year of high school. I was always taught to ignore pain so that I could either earn starting positions on the football team or keep from being replaced, honestly living with pain was a way of life for those that play football and any sport for that matter.

The first time I had experienced back pain was my junior year of high school while sitting in class, I felt like I was being stabbed in the middle of my back with a dull knife. The pain was so severe that I asked my teacher could I lay on my back on the cold floor during class, strangely enough my teacher allowed me to do so and I must say I did experience some relief and was able to attend football practice later that afternoon. Some of you reading this may ask yourself why didn't I go to the school nurse, doctor or notify my parents? Like I said before, we were taught to do anything to stay on the field and we had the mindset that some pain was to be expected. I was just un-aware that this back pain would resurface multiple times throughout my adulthood with each occurrence being more severe than the last.

    I should also be honest about other factors behind my reasoning for avoiding seeking professional help. One major reason being is that my family was poor at best and I did not want to be a burden financially to my mother which was my sole supporter. Another reason for not seeking medical attention was that I had a fear of visiting doctor's especially regarding a potential back injury mainly due to mis-information from those around me. Nevertheless, failure to act on my part resulted in my back problems not only progressing but also having a major impact on my life. It is my hope that this short book will not only help others to bounce back from back injuries that result in surgery, but also help those that have apprehensions about seeking medical advice to do so.

Chapter 1: The Signs

There were several signs that periodically alerted me to the fact that I had underlying back issues. The first sign was the incident in high school in which I had to lay on the floor in the back of a class room to alleviate severe pain. The next sign that I had back issues was during my high school graduation ceremony, I was struck with severe pain throughout my entire upper body, the pain was so severe that I could barely lift my arms. I thought that the pain was simply me being nervous about walking on stage in front of thousands of people, so I ignored it, the pain subsided within a day or 2. I managed to earn a scholarship to college where I would play collegiate football. I was pretty much pain free as far as my back was concerned all the way to my junior year, during my junior year I would have that familiar pain recur off and on that I had in high school. This pain would intensify each time it returned and eventually became so severe that I could not lift my arms above my head.

At this point with pain like this you would think I went to the doctor or at least my athletic training staff, wrong I continued to push through the pain. As I reflect on those days I realized that was a drastic mistake and I should have gotten medical aid. Instead of seeking medical attention I chose to self-medicate with alcohol. We see the commercials all the time about people battling addiction and many of them saying that their addictive habit started with some sort of pain. Well, I was no different from the individuals that I would see on the commercials. When pain would come I would drink alcohol until it went away. I dreamed of playing in the NFL and one thing I knew was certain, if a person had a bad medical report they had no chance at playing on the next level especially a guy from a small school. I am not going to make any excuses, I will simply say I didn't know any better and would soon learn from my mistakes.

I manage to continue to hide the pain throughout my senior year of college, but my athletic performance began to deteriorate, I ran slower and became a body that just got in the way because of pain. My teammates will most likely tell you that I was a great offensive lineman that always played very well I was a good football player, however I also know when I was limited and how much better I could have been. By this time my dream of going to the NFL subsided, not because I didn't have the talent or at least feel I had the talent, but because I knew there was something wrong with me and there was no way I could perform on that level. I would go on to graduate college and begin to work, the pain would continue to come back of and on but this time it would last for months. Alcohol was no longer working to keep the pain at bay and by this time because I was working I had health insurance. so I went to see a doctor.

Before I go further I would like to add though I was an overweight offensive lineman I didn't begin to have high blood pressure until my junior year of college and each year it would get higher. I contributed my high blood pressure to alcohol abuse, but I would learn later in life that my back/spinal issues caused my blood pressure to become elevated. Consider your blood pressure like a check engine light, doctors will often prescribe blood pressure medications to treat symptoms, but never attacking the underlying issues. Keep in mind it is also up to the patient to know his or her body and tell doctors everything.

Back to my story, eventually doctors would tell me that I had arthritis in my spine. The way I found out about the arthritis was due to being rear ended in a car accident, the doctors ordered a routine x-ray of the back which showed the arthritis. I'm not a doctor I do however have family members that have suffered with arthritis, to me it seemed like a legitimate diagnosis. Keep in mind by this time I had years of abuse to my body due to football, power lifting and martial arts, so an arthritis diagnosis was a no brainer to me. Eventually I would go a period of about 1 year in which I was not in so much pain. I decided to play some arena football when I was 26 years old, I manage to once again earn a starting position. I was no where near as good as I was in college, it felt as if I was running in mud. I can remember taking 3 to 5 Advil before every practice, so I could make it through. Arena football only lasted 1 year for me, I was physically incapable of playing. I honestly thought I had gotten too old and that stage of my life was simply over.

The stabbing pain would return, I would get medications prescribed to me such as pain killers and muscle relaxers that rarely did anything beside give me a stomach ache and make me sleepy. By this time the only athletic thing I could do was go to the gym and lift heavy weights, that would soon be over as well. Though I dealt with severe pain in my upper back I would lift weights, it seemed to be the only thing that caused some sort of relief. During training sessions, I would have little to no pain, but almost immediately after I would have intense pain. I was self-medicating at the local TGI-Fridays or whatever bar I could find at least 4 nights per week. I would have never thought that I would be an alcoholic pushing 30 years of age. This would go on for a couple of years until I hurt my low back in the gym, I suffered a herniated disc while doing a reverse hack squat with extremely heavy weight. This injury was the straw that broke the camels back and enough was enough.

I experienced just about every symptom one could think of that comes with a herniated disc from sciatica, numb legs and weakness. The symptoms had gotten so severe that I could barely walk under my own power which caused me to seek out a specialist. I went to see a specialist and he of course ordered an MRI on my lumbar spine which showed a herniated L4/L5 disc. Here is where I began to lose faith in the ability of doctors, the specialist told me that my issue was minor and there was nothing to worry about. He wrote a prescription for physical therapy and pain management which were both very costly and unproductive. The funny thing is that I told that specialist about all the pain I had in my upper back which I would later find out is the thoracic spine, he ignored me and treated me like I was just another number. Here you have a guy standing in front of you that has explained everything to you and you simply say don't worry and don't at least order imaging for the entire spine it is important for you the reader to know that this was the year 2011 not 1980. Now I am not a doctor, but that just doesn't appear to be best practice.

Chapter 2: Less Than Weak

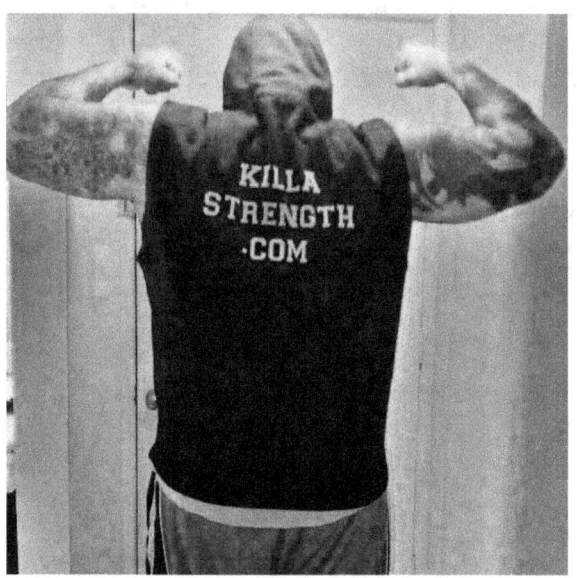

Since I was mis-diagnosed and told that I didn't need surgery I began to do my own research regarding recovering from a herniated disc. I tried everything from stretching to strengthening the area that was impacted which was the advice that I was given everywhere I looked. I even purchased expensive gym equipment that was supposed to help me strengthen and heal my injury. Nothing worked, I thought I had failed at rehabilitating myself and that I was just one of those unlucky people that would be damaged the rest of their lives. This type of epiphany is devastating and can take a major toll on one's life.

    Everything failed, it had gotten to the point that I could barely work and was afraid to go places due to my injury. I couldn't run, I couldn't walk for long periods of time, I couldn't sit for long periods of time and I couldn't lay on my back. I couldn't do anything, I felt that I may as well be in a wheelchair. Luckily for me things would get so severe that eventually I would have to have a second opinion. Due to circumstances out of my control I had to move back into the house with my mother and step-father trust me that alone is enough to make a person give up, I never thought I would have to move back in the house with my parents especially a college being a college graduate. Everything happens for a reason, things would get worse for me physically, but would also lead to the beginning of repairing the issues with my back.

During a conversation with my mother she asked me did I get a second opinion regarding my back, I told her no and she explained to me that many people are often mis-diagnosed just like me. So, I took her advice and sought out a second opinion. Armed with the same bad information I go from the previous doctor I explained to my doctor what my symptoms were and what I had been doing trying to remedy them. The doctor ordered tests, reviewed them and agreed that I needed to have the surgery especially if they were causing these types of issues. The surgery to be done was a microdiscectomy on my L4 and L5 discs.

Needless to say. I was excited to have found a surgeon that agreed that my symptoms were extreme and I needed to have the issue fixed. No less than one week after scheduling my surgery I ended up in an emergency room with severer tremors in both my legs. It was in the emergency room that the doctor explained to me that my symptoms were being caused by more than a l4 and l5 disc problems. The doctor ordered an emergency MRI for imaging of my entire spine, once I the imaging was complete I was immediately notified that I needed to have emergency surgery on my thoracic spine because bone from my spinal column had grown into the nerve root and was causing severe damage. Basically, when the bones grow into the nerves of the spinal column they restrict blood flow to the nerve, the nerve can't send the proper signals to the muscles and the nerve begins to die.

Spinal Surgery Timeline:

1. 2013 Thoracic Laminectomy T3, 4, 5, 8, 9, 10, 11

2. 2017 Microdiscectomy L4/L5/S1

3. 2018 Thoracic Laminectomy T6 & T7

Chapter 3: Surgery #1

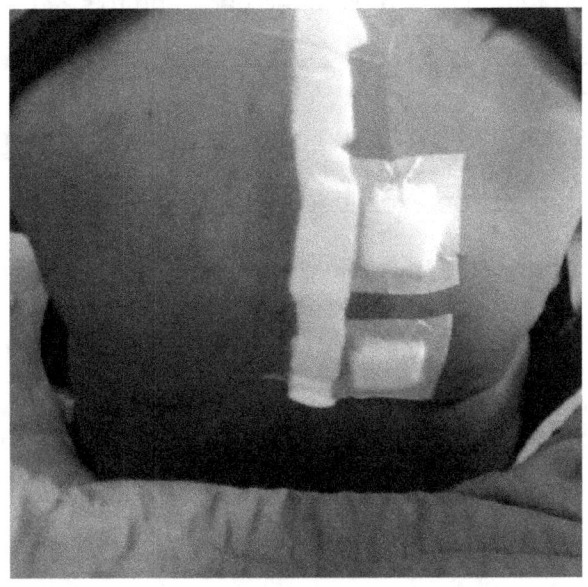

My surgery was done the next day, the surgery was a thoracic laminectomy on my thoracic spine in which the doctor uncapped the nerve root on levels t3, t4, t5, t6, t10 and t11. After surgery I was awakened by the anesthesiologist and the first thing I did was wiggle my toes without being prompted to by the tech, honestly it was something I saw on a television show as a kid. I could see my toes moving but I had little to no feeling in my legs and feet. I was a bit taken back and to say I was afraid of not being able to walk again was an understatement. The surgeon came in to speak with me the next morning and explained that due to the nerves being compressed in my spine for so long and the magnitude of the surgery it would take a very long time for me to regain full sensation and strength in my legs and there was also a possibility that I would not regain full use of my legs.

All I could hear while the surgeon was speaking that it would take time to heal and recover with complete disregard to the possibility that I may not have full use of my legs even after I am fully healed. I am a firm believer that we can control the outcomes of our lives especially when it comes to one's own body. I know that is a bold statement but keep in mind that is for those that still have some hope of a full recovery. After 2 days of laying in my hospital bed the hospital's physical therapists came in and got me up out of bed. Though I did not have much feeling in my legs I was able to walk with the assistance of holding on to someone. Though I was moving extremely slow this was a boost of confidence for me.

    I can not continue without telling you about the type of pain I was in, the pain literally felt like my back was ripped apart to my spine. I started out using a dilaudid while I was in the hospital to control the pain while I was in the hospital, the drug was so powerful that it had me in la la land, being a person that has never been high before this was a terrible feeling. Nevertheless, it was either control the pain with meds or suffer in agony. Once I was released (after 4 days) I was given, oxycodone, diazepam and some other pain killer I can't remember the name of. My first week at home I pretty much spent sitting on a couch in a drugged and depressed state. I literally had no idea what my future would hold let alone how I would get through this process.

You may be asking yourself what did he do for rehab/physical therapy? Well there is a funny story behind that. My insurance dropped my coverage immediately after my surgery therefore I was on my own regarding physical therapy. With no income and the social security administration refusing to give me disability I had no choice but to rehab myself. Luckily my years of athletics and personal training would pay off. I used the same philosophy that I used with building muscle and strength and that philosophy has always been to take baby steps all the way to the top. And so began the long challenging road to recovery.

Chapter 4: My First Self Rehab

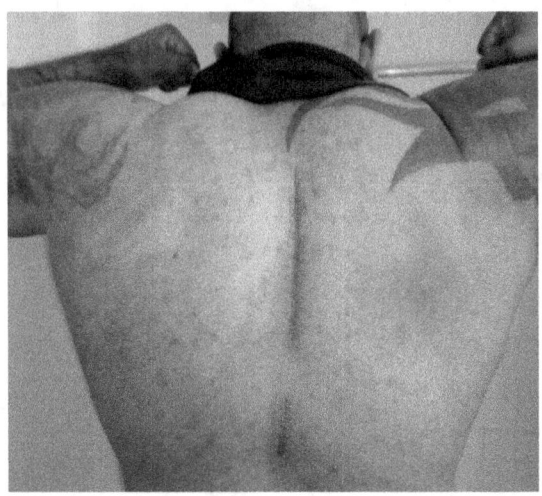

This chapter is more of a how to rehab yourself after a surgery similar to the surgery that I had myself. The first thing you need to know is that you are unique, no one has went through an identical situation as you have because it is flat out impossible for that to be the case. The next thing I will tell you is to do what you can and test your limits every day. You will fall, I mean that in the literal since of the word you will fall on your face, knees, buttock, back etc. Look at this as you would when a baby first learns to walk again, that's exactly what you yourself will be doing.

When I finally got off that reclining chair in my bedroom the first thing I did was to walk while using whatever was next to me to hold on to whether it was walls, chairs, tables etc. You see I refused to use a walker at the age of 29, I just couldn't bring myself to do so, I am not saying whether that was a good idea or not. I made it a point to get up and walk around at least 10 times per day no matter how severe my pain level was. After about a week I was no longer afraid to fall while walking and was able to start walking without grabbing on to walls. I would like to say that the numbness in my legs had subsided but that was not the case I had just gotten good at balancing myself due to constant practice.

Once I began to walk more consistently under my own power without the use of walls etc, I eventually started going to a local gym, I knew I couldn't do much but with controlled machines such as ellipticals and treadmills I could eventually improve my movement and balance even more. I started out walking very slow on level 1 on the treadmill for 20 to 30 minutes at a time due to my legs getting extremely tired after using them for extended periods of time. It's crazy to think that once I could play full football games, train hours of martial arts and never have the thought of my legs getting tired or failing me. This is a valuable lesson as well don't think about all the amazing things that you have done in the past just focus on the new challenge ahead of you. The more I thought about the things I used to be able to do prior to my injury the more depressed and discouraged I would become.

Not to get off topic but I have to say that mindset is of great importance, many of us say we believe in our abilities and positive outcomes until something bad comes along to truly test that faith. I won't get religious on you I will simply say that you have to believe in the things you can not see and be willing to put in the work to control your destiny when overcoming something like this. Everyday my faith was tested whether it was the falling, my legs getting tired etc., it was a constant test. The breakthroughs would come when I would lease expect it, an example of this is as simple as stepping on a curb, prior to my surgery I would get anxiety when it came to stepping-up on a 4-inch curb. I would stand and look at the curb for what felt like minutes before I would attempt to step up on to it, most of the time I would find a car to propel myself from.

Around a month had went by and I had eventually made my way to the elliptical and stairmaster, the treadmill no longer was a challenge. This brings me to another point I stated earlier, you must challenge yourself daily to test your boundaries and gauge your progress. Keep in mind at this point I still couldn't run or do things like lift heavy weights but I was getting better by the day. One thing that helped my progress was daily physical activity, it was very similar to that of a person with arthritis if I would stop or miss a day it felt as if my progress was reversing. Still being my first rehab, I am sure there were a million things I did wrong, one for sure I know was diet as well as different forms of exercise that may have then accelerated my rehabilitation. I will get to the other exercises as well as the best diet that worked for me later on in this short book, keep in mind I went through 3 back surgeries before I developed a solid rehab and diet regimen.

A few months would pass, I begin to lift weights again, I couldn't stay away from the weights I had developed what is now known as the dad bod and it made me physically ill to look at myself in the mirror. I just could then and will not subscribe to the idea of being "half the man I used to be", many have asked me why I continue to lift weights after going through surgeries like this, the truth is my first back problem stemmed from spinal stenosis which I was born with, the second stemmed from working on a sit down job for years destroying my low back and the 3 injury as you will read later had nothing to do with anything I have done and could not be avoided. I began to get strong again and had by this time been able to do just about everything in the gym even jump rope.

Though I seemed to be recovering quite nicely there were some mistakes I was making while rehabbing myself, I honestly didn't know the how small things in my life were affecting my health especially my back health. During this time-period I had gotten too comfortable and begin to revert to bad eating habits and the use of alcohol. Gradually my use and abuse of alcohol would increase but I didn't notice because I had yet become disciplined and focused enough. I will explain in detail in a later chapter how the foods we consume and things like alcohol effect our spine health. Nevertheless, I would soon start to decline again, it took a few years but slowly I would notice myself getting weaker, losing balance and having strange sensations in my legs and hips.

Chapter 5: Back Surgery #2

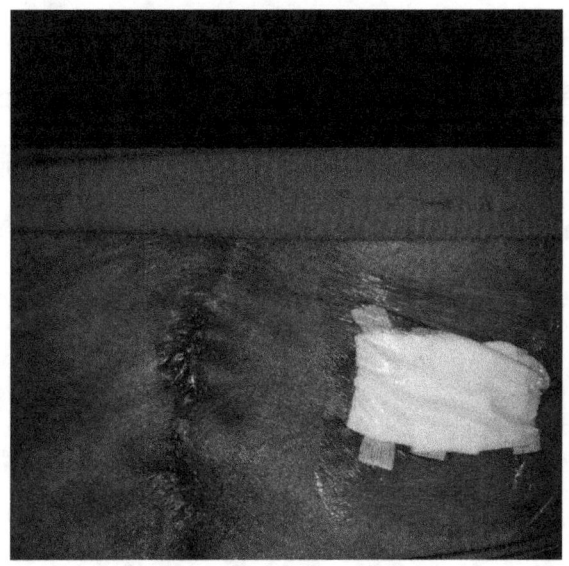

As my condition would begin to deteriorate over the course of the next 3 years I did little to stop the constant declination of my condition. Though I knew something was wrong I wasn't sure weather it was my previous L4/L5 issue that had yet to be resolved or if it was simply that my condition would not get better. I would find myself missing the gym due to pain in my lower back, the pain would keep me from standing upright and it would also cause different problems in other areas of my body. I would have hip pain and tightness that would prevent me from walking, my right foot began to turn inward while walking without me being able to keep it straight. While sleeping at night I would have mini tremors in my back, the tremors were so powerful that it felt as if my spine was shifting.

I would continue to deal with the issues happening, I had convinced myself that I was having these issues because I was working another desk job.

The job I was in at the time I would sit for no less that 4-hour periods straight because I was studying for a complicated financial service license. An important point I would like to make is that self-diagnosis can be a killer. It is important that when we have medical issues no matter how small we may think they are to consult a qualified physician that can diagnose and treat the issue. Small things tend to mount up, look at my situation with each issue I began to have there was a trickle-down effect until I was in worse shape than I had been in before. Some of you may think it idiotic that I ignored what was going on with my health, the only excuse I have is that I was uncertain, discouraged and flat out afraid that I was doomed to face these issues forever.

I did not make the conscious decision to visit an orthopedic surgeon until one day while lifting with a friend in the gym both my legs went numb. This was a feeling that was all too familiar to me, the filling was as if I was walking barefoot through quicksand. I thought maybe I had pinched a nerve or something due to the issues I already had with my low back, after all I did have the low back pain and the symptoms I mentioned previously. The numb feeling would not get better it was constant for at least a two-month period, I wanted to give the injury time to heal itself. I had no choice but to go to the doctor and get evaluated to see what was now causing my problem. I met with a good spine surgeon that ordered imaging for my back. After getting the imaging it appeared that my fears that my low back was causing my issues had come true.

The results from the latest MRI would show that my L4 and L5 disc had gotten far worse and I had a new issue with my S1 disc. My new spinal surgeon believed that everything that I was experiencing was due to the issues that had worsened within my lower back. Once again, I would go under the knife with hopes to finally rid myself of these debilitating issues, by this time I was 35 years of age and living the life of a 65-year-old due to my physical limitations. I would go on to have my surgery which based on my surgeon's opinion was a success. I didn't really know what to expect during my recovery, I just knew I would take it easy and heal the right way. Once again, I would have full control of my legs and it also appeared that the issue with my hip and foot were slightly better. I was very excited that I was finally fixed, I would no longer have these life limiting issues I had for so long.

Though I was healing something seemed to be off, I couldn't put my finger on the issue, but it felt like I was healing a bit too slow. With my first spinal surgery relief seemed to come faster, with this one it was like I was making small progress a little bit at a time. I would consult with my doctor and try an oral steroid that would hasten my recovery by reducing what my doctor and I thought were the side effects of inflammation. After taking my first course of the oral steroid I noticed relief, I had once again regained a significant amount of feeling in my legs. No less than a week after I finished my course of oral steroids I began to have the same symptoms, this time the symptoms would return any time that I would lay on my back whether it was in bed or elsewhere. My primary doctor insisted that I should try a couple more cycles of the oral steroid to see if that would fix my issues.

My condition had improved a lot or so I thought, I wasn't doing much beside going to work and sleeping. I wasn't lifting weights and I was avoiding all social events, I had a constant fear that my symptoms would return. Eventually I would develop the confidence to return to the gym, I would avoid any exercise in which I had to lay on my back because I was afraid that my symptoms would then return. Slowly but surely, I got more and more confident with my training and began to test those boundaries again. I began to use the smith machine for incline bench pressing and low and behold every time I would work over 200lbs my symptoms would return. It was obvious that something wasn't right, and I needed to see what was going on, maybe I was expecting too much too fast or I was simply doing something wrong with my recovery causing me to re-injure myself. My family and friends would always blame me for my injure, they would often say things like I lifted too many weights, I went to the gym too much and I was constantly injuring myself. With all these negative influences they were not helping the situation and honestly my doctors both that had done my surgeries did not contribute weightlifting, football nor martial arts to my injuries in fact they believed that my upper back issues stemmed from being born with a narrow spinal column and my bad low back was most likely caused by working desk jobs and sitting for long periods of time.

Back to my story, I set up a new appointment with my spinal doctor and he ordered new imaging fearing that my last surgery was not he success that he thought it was. The MRI was ordered, and the results were in, my low back looked perfect and I had not done anything to re-injure myself, my doctor recommended that I continue to rehab myself and monitor my progress. I was a tad bit discouraged with this new test results, I once again began to believe that maybe I would not live a normal life again and that sucks. The depression and self-doubt had begun to take its toll on me and my everyday life, I had become a negative person and some what of a recluse I simply was not someone in great spirits. I would continue to rehab myself and research things that may help with my recovery, google university is a great place to find tons of free information regarding almost any topic. This is where I discovered natural remedies for inflammation such as turmeric, ginger, fish oil and the things in one's diet that may cause back issues to worsen. I guess one could say that each issue we are faced with in life gives us the chance to re-evaluate and educate ourselves so that we can not only help ourselves but others along the way during our self-evolution.

    I began to rid my diet of sugars, vegetable oils, fried foods, alcohol and many other things that were quietly affecting my spinal health. I must say that my quality of life had improved. I generally felt better health wise but as far as my back it didn't appear to be improving in fact reducing the inflammation in my body seemed to be allowing me to pinpoint pain that I didn't know I had. After about a month of consuming turmeric daily I noticed that my back had begun to hurt where I had my first surgery. The pain was all too familiar I began to fear that the stenosis had struck again, but how could this be? I took pain pills and dealt with the pain for about two weeks, yes this was very stupid I should have went to the doctor. The pain had gotten so severe that I had to sleep on the floor which seemed to give me some relief, this was short-lived I slept on the floor for 2 nights and by the end of the second night I woke up with no feeling in my legs. This was horrible I thought I was paralyzed, I ended up in the emergency room where the doctors ordered an emergency MRI on my entire back. The pain was so severe the doctors had to give me strong pain medicine as well as pain killing patches affixed directly to my back. Laying on that MRI table I felt like I was going to die the pain felt as if I was laying on a mid-evil spike in the upper part of my back.

Chapter 6: Surgery #3

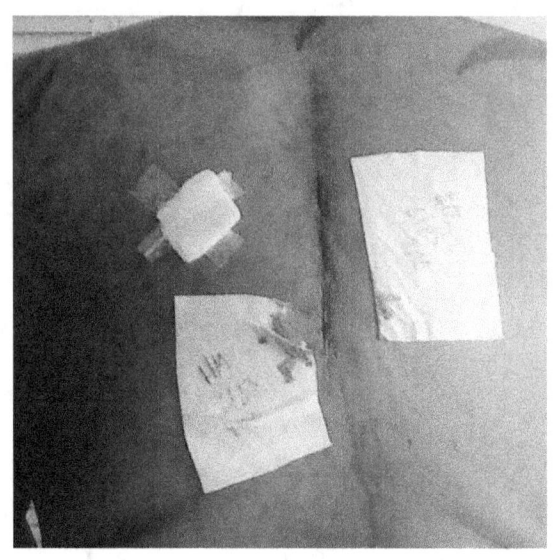

The results were in, the bones in my thoracic spine were growing into my spinal column and I was in danger of becoming paralyzed. I had a sick sense of relief because I now knew that I was not causing my spine to deteriorate. Apparently. this is something that is not un-common with spinal surgeries, when I had gotten my first surgery the surgeon skipped some spaces because my nerves were not pinched in those areas, what we didn't know is that my body would take those bones that had not been touched and cause theme to grow into the areas in which I had the nerves uncapped. This was a freak occurrence that does not happen to everyone but of course it did happen to me.

My spinal surgeon immediately scheduled surgery for the next day, I was relieved I truly believed that he would fix the problem once and for all and I would now make a full recovery. Once the surgery was completed I was told that it was a complete success. Something felt different, nothing felt off, I wasn't concerned that I wouldn't recover. This time I knew I had the chance to become my normal self again well honestly a new and better version of what I once was. Armed with my new-found knowledge of how the body works and the natural remedies available to treat inflammation that I would beat this thing once and for all. My goal with this surgery was to give my health and appearance a complete overhaul, you see I had always been a heavier person walking around at 330lbs with high blood pressure and a less than attractive physiques. I wanted to prove to myself as well as others that even with all the physical adversity that I was faced with I could change my outcome and become better than what I was before.

Now knowing what to expect after going through so many back surgeries I knew I could handle almost anything being thrown at me. This time I decided to get physical therapy and push my rehab to the limits. I was physically drained from this last surgery and this time I had no choice but to use a walker, I didn't have a problem with this because when I went into surgery I was all but paralyzed. I knew that using the walker would be short-lived, I used that walker for about 2 weeks and was able to upgrade to a cane. I was very week and my legs had very low reactions to stimulus. Luckily for me during this time I lived in an apartment complex where my unit was on the third floor, this was good for me because I would walk up and down the steps holding on to the rails to strengthen my legs and gain endurance. I documented all of this so that I could monitor my progression.

My latest strategy along with an excellent spinal surgeon has allowed me to regain a bit of my life back. I can honestly without a doubt in my mind say that this last surgery was a complete success. I am not 100% yet but I am on already far more ahead than I have been in years. Next, I will outline some of my training techniques as well as the dietary and lifestyle changes that continue to help me with my rehabilitation and body transformation.

Chapter 7: Dietary Changes

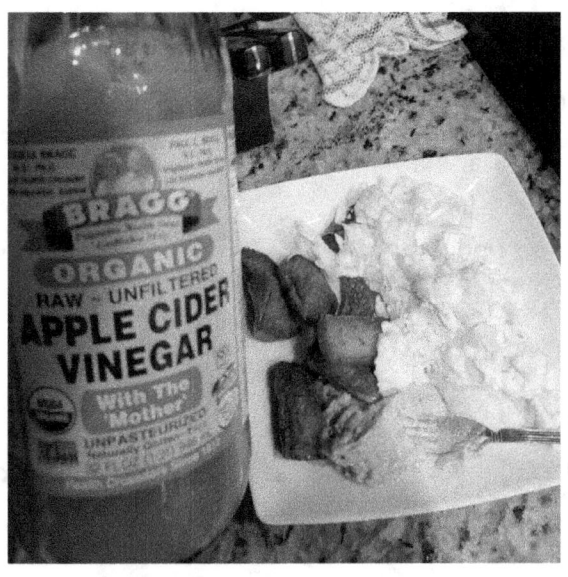

As I stated before that I not only changed my diet for the purposes of relieving inflammation but also for the purpose of transforming my physique into one that is more aesthetically pleasing. In this chapter I will outline the foods that I have omitted from my diet and also discuss why I removed them as well as the foods I have added and how they contribute to my ultimate goal. Keep in mind this is what has worked for me and everyone's situation is different, someone that has never been over weight or doesn't have an issue with things like high-blood pressure my not need to completely overhaul his or her diet.

Bread and Other Process Foods: Inflammatory Foods

The first food that I removed from my diet are processed carbohydrates such as bread, pasta, potato chips etc. These types of foods convert quickly into sugar which foster fat storage and create inflammation throughout the body beginning in the gut. Growing up and throughout adult hood I would eat bread with every meal I had no knowledge of how this type of food would impact my health as well as physical appearance. Below I will list three things that you should know about bread, though there are many and the list could go on for pages I felt these were the essential top three that you should know.

1. Bread (whole grain/wheat): The grains are broken down into refined powders which causes the body to rapidly absorb it, ironically bread can be just as bad or worse than consuming some candy bars. The sugar spike not only leads to inflammation, but it also increases fat deposits, increases risk for high blood pressure and can also cause things like acne.
2. Gluten: Most breads contain gluten many individuals can't tolerate gluten and have issues with their digestive tract as a result. This is important to understand because poor digestion decreases the amount of nutrients absorbed into the body from food causing the body to not

heal efficiently as well as cause obesity and malnutrition.

3. Bread is also a poor choice in one's diet because it is low in essential nutrients, again to heal and function properly one must choose nutrient dense foods that help the body repair itself.

Conclusion: Though bread is very tasty and is served with virtually everything we eat here in the U.S. it can be dangerous do to it's ingredients and the way it converts into sugar. Bread is bad whether you are recovering from an injury such as me or you just want to be a healthy person with a nice physique.

The next food that I have eliminated from my diet is all processed foods, to keep it simple I like to use this definition when determining what foods are processed and what foods are not "Food processing is the transformation of cooked ingredients, by physical or chemical means into food, or of food into other forms. Food processing combines raw food ingredients to produce marketable food products that can be easily prepared and served by the consumer". Let's take a deeper look, processed foods typically contain preservatives whether it be sodium, sugars or chemicals that are hard to pronounce, processed foods are an enemy to general health the sodium in these foods alone can have adverse effects on one's kidneys, liver even heart. Here in the United States our foods tend to have more sodium and sugar than other countries, I guess this is contributed to us being a part of a highly capitalistic society.

Sugar or what I like to call Pointless Poison

Many processed foods have labels that state natural, healthy etc. One must understand that the labels can be deceiving, it is imperative that we look at the ingredients and the amount of servings recommended for those type of products if we choose to consume them. Below I will list the health risks of processed foods.

1. Sugar and High Fructose Corn Syrup: In 2018 we all know or should know that sugar has no nutritional value and yields virtually no positive effects on the human body. High sugar consumption can lead to insulin resistance, increased fat accumulation, harmful cholesterol and high triglycerides. Again, this simply put means that sugar consumption does not just make a person fat but also effects other areas of the body.

2. Processed foods are enhanced by manufactures so that people like you and I can consume as much as possible which means buy as much as possible. Simply put the foods are designed to taste damn good and for you to not only enjoy consuming them but also crave them.
3. Processed Food Causes Addiction: Because these foods are enhanced and designed to want more many individuals find it difficult to stop consuming them.
4. Processed Foods are High in Refined Carbohydrates: Bread isn't the only enemy to your body, many of the processed foods we consume are loaded with the same ingredients you will find in bread and in some cases larger amounts.

This is because refined carbohydrates have such a close relationship to sugar that they also become highly addictive.

Conclusion: processed foods are a great product for manufacturers to make money due to their addictiveness. Though I doubt that manufacturers have some sinister plan to make people sick it is fair to say that they want you to be addicted to their foods so that you can buy more, it is just unfortunate that many individuals don't understand the ill effects on the human body from the ingredients in these so-called foods. Again, consuming the correct healthy foods is essential for a healthy body especially someone dealing with back surgery.

Alcohol: The most dangerous and readily available drug

The next food I eventually removed from my diet is Alcohol, I know you are saying alcohol isn't a food, but I would like to point out for the purposes of this book anything one consumes that contains calories is in fact a food. I know that saying alcohol is the most dangerous and readily available drug is somewhat of a bold statement. The fact is it is true alcohol is readily available and can be purchased by anyone over the age of 21. Alcohol has the same affects as opioids and other stimulants, it dulls sensitivity and decreases brain function, these are common side effects we all know about. Many of us have a mis-understanding of alcohol consumption guidelines, most individuals consume alcohol in dangerous amounts weekly and are completely un-aware of its impact on their overall health. Below I will list the damaging effects of alcohol as it pertains to rehabilitating a spinal injury as well as a bit of info regarding recommended consumption, I must admit I am a bit biased in my opinion based on my personal and familial history with alcohols devastating effects on one's health.

1. Excessive alcohol consumption can cause disc desiccation, a more familiar name would be degenerative disc disease. Degenerative disc disease generally rears its head with an aging spine, could excessive alcohol consumption age one's spine?
2. Osteoarthritis which can be extremely painful can occur do to excessive alcohol consumption.

3. Weight gain is an obvious but subtle side effect of excessive alcohol consumption. Like it or not the spine is affected by changes in weight. Extra weight places undo stress on the spine which can cause several problems.

Alcohol Consumption Guidelines

Many people mis-understand what one drink means, here is an overview of the definition of one drink: One drink is defined as 12 fluid ounces of beer (5% alcohol), 5 fluid ounces of wine (12% alcohol), or 1.5 ounces of 80 proof (40% alcohol) distilled spirits/liquor. One drink contains 0.6 fluid ounces of alcohol. Binge drinking is defined as consuming 4-5 drinks within a 2 hour-period depending on if you are male or female. Here is the confusion most people count drinks as the number of drinks that they have, the reality is that drinking is based on units and not how many glasses, cups or bottles you have. One martini is 5 units of alcohol meaning if you drink 1 and that's just 1 martini you are now binge drinking. It is important for individuals to understand this because health risks from alcohol consumption increase when one begins to binge drink. Who has just one martini? Ask yourself, have you ever woke up with back pain after a night of drinking or a few drinks? It is not your imagination alcohol is affecting your spine.

Do your own research regarding alcohol and your spine, alcohol has no therapeutic effects on the human body. Ironically while writing this book I discovered that alcohol even in small uses such a wine do not have a positive effect on the heart as we were all once told. It never was the alcohol itself that helped the heart it was the antioxidants in the fruit that is used to make some wines that is good for the heart. Why not just eat fruit?

Dairy Products: A hidden ingredient that causes inflammation

Removing Dairy products may also help you alleviate inflammation, there is an ingredient in dairy milk called casein which is notorious for causing inflammation. Butter, cheese and creams should be removed. It is important to understand that vitamin d is great for strong bones, the processing of dairy products makes many of the products bad for you especially if you are dealing with rehabbing a painful back injury or you simply want to obtain the optimal physique. If you can find high quality raw milk you can consume that with no issues. One should also consider exposure to direct sunlight and if that doesn't work there are plenty of legitimates supplements that can provide a significant amount of vitamin D. Of all the foods I have omitted from my diet I will say that dairy caused me the least problems physically, with so many options such as raw milk, fat free milk and low sugar milk I have been able to consume a sufficient amount of vitamin D daily.

Conclusion: For me omitting many of these foods has done wonders for not only my recovery, but my overall health as well. From cholesterol to blood pressure I am in much better health over all at the age of 36 versus my health in my 20's. It is imperative to understand that no one is perfect this type of regiment is not easy to keep up with especially if you like me have been given the wrong dietary information your entire life. My advice is to take it one day at a time and keep in mind this is a lifestyle that will help you to not only repair your injury but help you live a better quality of life over all. Being more fit in general will have a huge impact on your social and economic life, clothing costs, food costs, medical expenses and even the cost of health and life insurance goes down when one is healthy not too mention you tend to save money because you are purchasing far less junk.

Foods and Supplements to Add

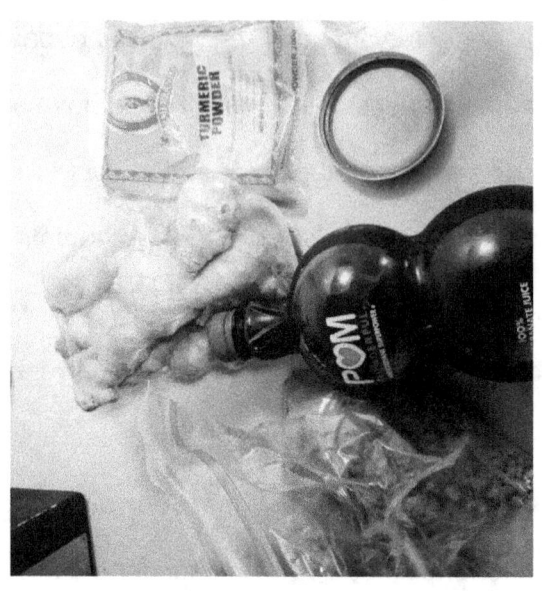

In this next chapter I will discuss some of the foods I have added to my diet that have helped me along with my recovery and my health.

- Turmeric- reduces inflammation, kills viruses, loaded with nutrients. Turmeric can prevent cancer by stopping cellular growth. Turmeric alleviates arthritis. Turmeric helps with diabetes. Turmeric reduces cholesterol. Turmeric is a natural immune booster. Turmeric helps clean and heal wounds. Turmeric helps break down fat which aids in weight loss. Turmeric helps with digestion by lessoning bloating and gas. Turmeric prevents liver disease. I can personally attest to the benefits of turmeric, I consume it in both the root and powder form. I typically put the root in a blender with water.

- Ginger- relieves nausea, digestive issues and pain due to its phenolic compounds. Ginger reduces inflammation. Ginger may reduce the risk of heart disease in those that suffer with type two diabetes due to reducing the amount of sugar in blood. Ginger may lower cholesterol levels. Ginger may improve brain function. I typically mix the ginger with the turmeric.

- Beets- reduces blood pressure. Beets prevent certain cancers (skin, lung and colon). Beets boost energy levels due to the naturally occurring carbohydrates. Beets improve sexual performance, due to boron. Beets improve mental health due to the betalains. Beets cleanse the digestive tract which reduce inflammation.
- Omega 3 Fish Oil: causes weight loss do to improved digestion function, reduction in body fat storage and decreases appetite. Fish oil aids in better heart health reducing triglyceride levels. Improves mood by improving the release

of serotonin alleviating inflammation in the brain. Fish oil improve vison. Fish oil fights inflammation throughout the body. I typically take fish oil in the morning and before bedtime.

- White Rice: white rice is cholesterol free and sodium free. White rice is gluten free and non-allergenic. White rice prevents and treats gastrointestinal distress. White rice is good for heart health by lowering cholesterol levels when replacing processed carbohydrates. White rice is easier to absorb, digest and excrete compared to brown rice. White rice can boost organs metabolic activities. White rice boosts muscle growth.

Conclusion: As you can see the list of foods and supplements that I have added is not very lengthy however each food and supplement is packed with health benefits. To fully recover from surgeries such as mine one must be in optimal physical condition and to do so one must consume the right foods. As you can see I am not promoting going to the local nutrition store and buying a bunch of supplements, the majority of what you need can be found at your local grocery store. When purchasing a supplement such as fish oil it is important that you do your own research as to the purity of the product, due to a loosely regulated supplement industry it can be difficult to find pure product.

Chapter 8: Get Physical

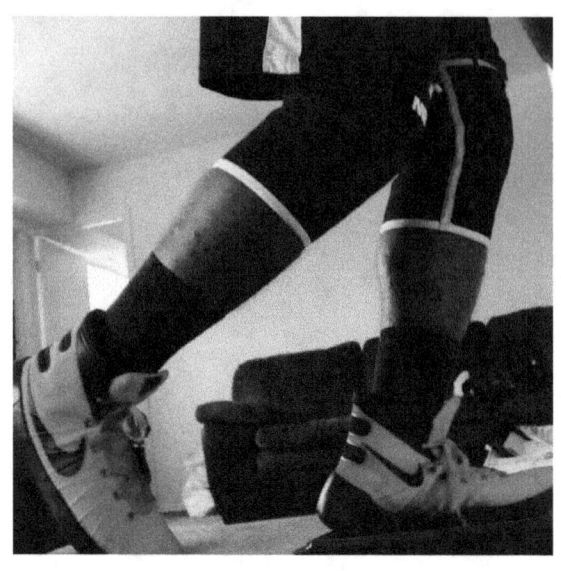

It is important to understand that you will not get healthier nor regain your quality of life if you don't exercise. I understand that everyone's situation is unique, and everyone has different limitations whether it be physical or otherwise. What I will list in this chapter is the benefits of different types of physical activity as it pertains to spinal surgery rehabilitation and overall fitness. You have options that are available to you, always remember do what you can and push it daily. For each 2 of my surgeries I couldn't walk under my own power, I suffered with both atrophy and numbness it was a daunting task just attempting to walk. I understand all to well the physical and psychological toll these type of surgeries on a person. Being able to support your own bodyweight and maintain balance is the ability that many of us take for granted until we are not able to do those things without some sort of assistance or completely under our own power.

Sitting to Standing: One of the most difficult things to do after a spinal surgery is standing, between the pain from the surgery itself and the weakness of one's legs it is very difficult to stand under one's own power. With anything practice will make perfect, what I did after each surgery was to practice standing up and sitting down slowly multiple time per day. The easiest way to do this is to use a walker or place your hands on the back of a chair while using your hands to both propel and balance yourself as you sit and stand.

Though sitting and standing exercises will strengthen the muscles within the entire body there are many other benefits. This type of exercise can make bones in the legs stronger as well as strengthen the spine itself. You will also improve your circulation, it is important to understand that it is easy to develop blood clots within the legs and other areas after back surgery because many individuals simply are not mobile while improving circulation you will also notice a positive effect on blood pressure which is important because some of the post-surgery medications tend to have a negative effect on the blood pressure. Your respiration will also be improved because the diaphragm is less restricted which allows the lungs to function better. Muscles tend to tighten after back surgery which can make getting around even more difficult that it already is post-surgery, the sitting and standing exercises can aid in loosening those tight muscles. Sitting to standing also allows for improved digestion, this is highly important due to the fact some of the medicines you will be prescribed post-surgery will halt bowel function which leads to other issues.

This is one of the easiest available exercises you can do on your own, I will not lie to you, you will be frustrated, you will experience pain. The more consistent you become with these exercises the less pain you will experience and the quicker you will be able to walk under your own power. The easiest way to do this exercise starting out is in the morning when you first wake up using your bed because it will give you some spring upward when standing and a soft cushy landing while sitting and do the same at night, start with 3 sets of 10 reps and work your way up to 5 sets of 30 or more reps. If you can, have someone time you weekly to monitor your improvements.

Walking: Walking will have many of the same effects that you will experience with sitting to standing exercises such as better circulation, digestion and the strengthening of the muscles to help reverse or avoid atrophy. Because walking is a low impact exercise it can be ideal for one's recovery however everyone is not able to walk after spinal surgery which is why it was not first on my list for exercises. If you can walk immediately after your surgery, you will most likely be on the road to a speedy recovery. Since I had little to no feeling in my legs let alone balance I found the best way for me to walk was to use stairs with rails. Using the stairs while holding on to rails aloud me to gradually improve my leg strength while securing myself gripping the rails. I believe walking up and down steps several times a day aloud me to walk under my own power faster. My only advice is to take your time and take baby steps, try to add a little more everyday whether you are walking un-assisted or you are using a stairway with rails like I had to.

Core Strengthening: Core strengthening is highly important when rehabilitating a spinal injury for many reasons. The abdominal and back muscles support the spine which allow it to function properly and remain stable creating better bone structure. The main groups of muscle to be aware of when strengthening one's core are the Obliques/Rotators (these muscles are used to stabilize the spine when upright, they also help with rotating the spine which has an effect on posture. The Extensors/glute and back muscles (these muscles are used to straighten the back, extend and lift, and move the hip away from the body (abduct). Flexors/abdominal and iliopsoas muscles these muscles do everything from bend and support the spine from the front to control the arch of the lumbar spine and adduct the hip (move the thigh toward the spine).

Now that we know the key areas that contribute to the spine let's look at a few of the exercises that a person can do that has just underwent spinal surgery. It has been my experience that the least painful core exercise is stomach vacuuming exercises which strengthen the abdominal wall. As pain begins to subside and some stability returns the next step in the progression is planking which strengthen both the abdominal wall and the lower back. It took me a couple of months of these before I moved to more demanding exercises such as back extensions, leg raises and crunches. Depending on the severity of your surgery and the amount of weakness you have after surgery the decision is yours regarding which exercises to begin with. It is highly important that are aware of your incision, that car needs to heal before doing anything besides vacuuming exercises.

Take your time and work with your physician and physical therapist to see what core training regimen best suites you for your specific situation. I understand that some individuals may not have the luxury of physical therapy which was what I experienced with my first 2 spinal surgeries, if this is the case google is a great tool for beginning your abdominal strengthening regimen. Keep in mind you know your body better than anyone else and luckily, we live in an age where just about any information we need is right at our finger tips.

Returning to the gym: Here is where rehabilitation can get a bit tricky, if you were an athlete such as myself you may be familiar with the benefits of strength training and using a gym with all it's wonderful equipment to your full benefit. This can be both a gift and a curse, on the one hand the experienced gym goer may be fully aware of how to properly train and strengthen all areas of the body while on the other hand due to the back injury and the surgery one may not have the same physical capabilities as before and this can cause extreme anxiety. It is not uncommon to face both fear and anxiety as it relates to returning to normal activity especially the gym. I myself could barely hold myself up let alone lift a weight in the gym after my surgery. One has to start from scratch and take advantage of the things the gym can offer to help with healing, an example is cardiovascular equipment such as stationary bikes, treadmills, ellipticals and stair masters.

This type of equipment is great because it allows you to do more than you would if you were just walking outside or doing the sit to stand exercises. This is key because not only will the equipment allow you to maintain some healthy level of conditioning, but it will also allow you to progress and move forward with your rehab. Things will be hard at first, you may find yourself starting at level 1 for all equipment but that's ok. If you are consistent and push yourself a little more each day you will get closer and closer to your normal self and honestly starting from scratch may allow you to become a better version of yourself than previously before. As I mentioned earlier in this book, I was in poor health mainly because of a poor diet, alcohol abuse and I never did any cardio when I went to the gym. Now I am close to my original strength, I weigh over 50 pounds less, my health is better and I feel better about myself.

Eventually you will be cleared to begin to lift weights, weights can be scary after back surgery simply because in most cases the surgeons have cut through a lot of muscle to get through to the spine. When I was first cleared to lift weights I was very afraid, I thought that weight lifting somehow contributed to all of these injuries when the truth is the weight lifting actually delayed the progression of my back problems. This is the point where you really don't want to focus on the old you and what you could do before, now is the time to really learn your body and strengthen every aspect of it. Start with machines and lift very light, focus on activating your muscles and developing them properly. Progress at your own pace, you will eventually move back to the free weights. It is important to note that at one point you will be very weak however consistency will lead you back to where you were before your surgery my advice is to focus on small victories not past success.

Recovery from training: Once you become active again, walking, lifting weights etc you will find yourself taking 2 steps forward and sometimes 1 step back. When I say one step back I am speaking of symptoms returning such as pain, numbness, weakness etc. You will have days where your body feels as if there has been no progress and you have reinjured yourself. The reality is that after back surgery you will deal with swelling and scar tissue for a very long time, for this reason you will often have symptoms that were very similar to what landed you in the hospital in the first place. As you begin to kick up physical activity this will happen often, but each occurrence will be less severe.

It is of high importance that your use your anti-inflammatory medicines and muscle relaxers along with natural remedies such as the turmeric and ginger. Ice will also become your best friend the goal is to fight the inflammatory response from your surgery both internally and externally. Try to ice at least 3 times per day and avoid heat. Get plenty of rest, stay hydrated and stretch as often as possible. Know when to back off from the gym and training, if you find yourself in too much pain listen to your body, rest, stretch and EAT!

The ultimate goal is to get near where you used to be and that is going to take work!

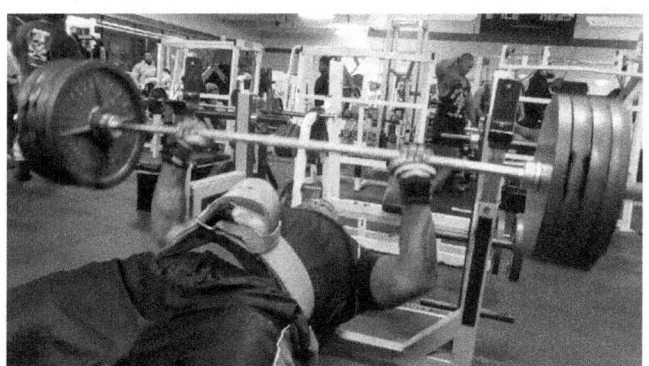

www.ingramcontent.com/pod-product-compliance
Lightning Source LLC
Chambersburg PA
CBHW052336220526
45472CB00001B/443